Table of Contents

A disorder of the central nervous system that affects movement, often including tremors.

Nerve cell damage in the brain causes dopamine levels to drop, leading to the symptoms of Parkinson's.

Parkinson's often starts with a tremor in one hand. Other symptoms are slow movement, stiffness and loss of balance.

Medication can help control the symptoms of Parkinson's.

BREAKFAST

1. Baked Mac and Cheese

Prep Time: 15Minutes

Cook Time: 1HR 5Minutes

Servings: 8

Ingredients:

- 1 lb. elbow macaroni
- 2–3 slices white bread, toasted
- 7 tablespoons butter, divided
- 2 tablespoons flour
- 1 12-ounce can evaporated milk
- 1/2 cup whole milk
- 1 teaspoon ground mustard
- 1 1/2 pounds cheddar cheese, grated
- 8 ounces American, Gruyere, or any other smooth melting cheese, grated or cut into chunks
- 2 eggs, beaten

Instructions

1. PREP: Preheat the oven to 375 degrees. Pour the macaroni into a large bowl and cover with hot water and stir in a big pinch of salt. Let the noodles soak for about 30 minutes while you prep the other ingredients.

2. BREADCRUMBS: Melt two tablespoons of the butter. Pulse the bread through a food processor, and add the butter. Set aside.

3. SAUCE BASE: Melt the butter in a large saucepan. Add the flour and cook, stirring constantly, until light golden blonde. Add the evaporated milk and whole milk, very slowly, whisking constantly to achieve a nice smooth, thick sauce. Stir in the mustard. Bring to a simmer over medium heat. Remove from heat to add the cheeses – stir until melted. Season to taste.

4. GET READY TO BAKE: Whisk about a cup of sauce with the eggs in a separate bowl (to increase the temperature of the eggs gradually). Once combined, add that egg mixture in with the rest of the sauce. Add the drained macaroni and stir to combine. Pour into a greased rectangular or square baking dish.

5. BAKE: Top with the breadcrumbs, cover with foil, and bake for 30 minutes. Remove foil and bake for another 5 minutes to get the breadcrumbs toasty and nice.

Serve with salt, pepper, hot sauce, or whatever you like with your baked mac and cheese.

Prep Time: 15 Minutes

Cook Time: 35 Minutes

Servings: 6

Ingredients:

Salad:

- 1 butternut squash, peeled and cubed (about 3 cups)
- 1 can Dakota's Pride Garbanzo Beans, rinsed and drained
- a drizzle of oil
- 1 teaspoon kosher salt
- 2–3 cloves garlic
- 4–5 cups Simply Nature Organic Chopped Kale
- 1 honeycrisp apple, sliced
- 1/2 cup Southern Grove Pepitas
- 1/2 cup Southern Grove Dried Cherries

Dressing:

- 1/2 cup olive oil
- juice of 1 lemon
- 1/2 teaspoon salt (more to taste)

- black pepper to taste
- 1 tablespoon sugar

Instructions

1. Roast: Preheat the oven to 425 degrees. Place squash and chickpeas on a sheet pan. Drizzle with oil, sprinkle with salt. Place garlic cloves in the center of a small piece of foil. Drizzle with oil and fold it up into a little packet. Place the packet on the sheet pan. Roast everything for 30-40 minutes.
2. Dressing: Whisk the oil, lemon juice, salt, pepper, and sugar together. When the sheet pan comes out of the oven, mash up the roasted garlic and add it to the dressing.
3. Kale: In a large bowl, drizzle the kale with a little bit of dressing (hello, flavor!). Massage it – as in, just, like, squeeze it – until it's deep green and the texture has relaxed a little bit. This just makes it more tender and pleasant to eat.
4. Salad: Place kale in a large salad bowl. Top with squash and chickpeas. Arrange little fanned-out apple slices on the salad (pretty!). Dot the whole thing with pepitas and dried cherries, and finish with the rest of the

dressing. Serve warm or cold! IT'S A BEAUTIFUL
MASTERPIECE.

Prep Time: 25 Minutes

Cook Time: 35 Minutes

Servings: 4

Ingredients:

Roasted Herbed Squash:

- 1 butternut squash, peeled and diced, + olive oil and salt
- 1 teaspoon Simply Nature Organic Thyme Leaves
- 1 small onion, thinly sliced
- Maple Mustard Brussels with Walnuts and Cherries:
- 1 package brussels sprouts, trimmed and cut + olive oil and salt
- 1/2 cup Southern Grove Walnuts
- 1/2 cup Southern Grove Dried Cherries
- 2 tablespoons Specially Selected 100% Pure Maple Syrup
- 2 tablespoon olive oil
- 1 teaspoon Dijon mustard
- Creamy Garlic Mashed Potatoes:

- 1 1/2 pounds round potatoes + olive oil and salt
- 6 cloves garlic, + olive oil and wrapped in foil
- 1/4 cup Countryside Creamery Salted Butter
- 1/4 cup broth or milk
- 1/4 cup Friendly Farms Sour Cream
- kosher salt to taste (I used about 1 teaspoon)

Instructions

1. Roasting Everything: Preheat oven to 425 degrees. Place squash and potatoes + seasonings on a sheet pan or roasting pan. Place brussels sprouts + seasonings on a sheet pan or roasting pan, cut side down. Roast squash and potatoes for 15 minutes. Add brussels sprouts to the oven; roast both pans another 20-30 minutes. During the last 5-or-so minutes, add the walnuts and cherries to the brussels sprout pan to get them nice and toasty.

Prep Time: 10Minutes

Cook Time: 50Minutes

Servings: 12

Ingredients:

Apple Cake:

- 1 1/2 cups brown sugar
- 1/3 cup oil
- 1 egg
- 1 cup buttermilk or (1 cup milk + 1 tablespoon white vinegar)
- 1 teaspoon vanilla
- 1 teaspoon baking soda
- 2 1/2 cups flour
- 2 1/2 cups chopped apples (see notes)

Cinnamon Sugar Topping:

- 1/2 cup sugar
- 1 teaspoon cinnamon
- 1 tablespoon butter, melted

Instructions

1. Preheat oven to 325 degrees. Mix or whisk ingredients in order given, stirring until just combined. Fold in your apples.

2. Pour batter into a buttered 9×13 pan (alternatively, you can line with parchment paper).

3. Combine last 3 ingredients to make a topping and sprinkle / spread it evenly over the batter.

4. Bake for 45 minutes. Test with a toothpick if needed. Serve with honey butter or whipped cream if you want. APPLE CAKE IS THE BEST!

Prep Time: 10Minutes

Cook Time: 30Minutes

Servings: 6

Ingredients:

Simple Delicious Tomato Sauce:

- 2 tablespoons olive oil
- quarter of an onion, minced
- 1 large clove garlic, minced or thinly sliced
- 12 ounces DeLallo Passata Tomato Purée
- 1/2 cup broth or water
- torn basil
- 1/4 cup mascarpone cheese
- 1/2 teaspoon salt

Gnocchi:

- one 16-ounce package DeLallo Potato Gnocchi (I used shelf-stable gnocchi but frozen would also work)
- a handful of baby spinach
- 8 ounces fresh mozzarella cheese slices
- Parmesan cheese

Instructions

1. Make the sauce: Preheat oven to 400 degrees. Heat the olive oil over medium low heat. Add the onion and garlic; sauté until translucent and fragrant. Add passata and water or broth; bring to a low simmer. Add torn basil, mascarpone, and salt. YUM.

2. Bake it up: Add gnocchi and spinach. Stir to coat evenly with sauce. Top with mozzarella slices and a sprinkle of Parmesan. Bake for 15-20 minutes, until gooey and light golden brown on top. Serve with more basil. THE END. That's it. You're in heaven.

Prep Time: 5 Minutes

Cook Time: 15 Minutes

Servings: 5

Ingredients

- Lettuce Wraps
- olive oil
- One 14-ounce block extra firm tofu – minimally pressed to remove water
- about 2 cups cooked brown rice and/or quinoa or other grains – I use the 8.5 ounce precooked packages so it's very, very easy
- butter lettuce or leaf lettuce for wrapping
- spicy mayo (see notes)
- chopped peanuts or crispy onions for topping
- SOS Peanut Sauce
- 1/2 cup teriyaki sauce
- juice of 1 orange
- 1/4 cup peanut butter
- a squirt of Sriracha or other chile sauce if you want

Instructions

1. Cook the tofu: Heat a few swishes of oil in a nonstick skillet over medium high heat. Add the tofu and crumble in the pan. Cook until slightly browned. While that's cooking, whisk up all sauce ingredients in a bowl.

2. Add rice and sauce: Add the rice and most of the sauce to the pan. Sauté for 5 minutes or so – just enough to get some browning / light caramelization and get everything nice and yummy. Season with salt to taste.

3. Fill and serve: Spoon your tofu and brown rice filling into crispy little pieces of lettuce. Top with something crunchy (peanuts? crispy onions?) and something creamy (spicy mayo all the way) and drizzle with a little extra sauce, and now tell me this isn't your favorite meal of the week.

Prep Time: 15 Minutes

Cook Time: 45 Minutes

Servings: 6

Ingredients:

For the Instant Pot:

- 5 medium carrots, chopped
- 5 stalks celery, chopped
- half of an onion, chopped
- 3 cloves garlic, minced
- 1 cup uncooked wild rice
- 8 ounces fresh mushrooms, sliced
- 4 cups vegetable or chicken broth
- 1 teaspoon salt
- 1 teaspoon poultry seasoning
- 1/2 teaspoon dried thyme

For the Stovetop:

- 6 tablespoons butter
- 1/2 cup flour
- 1 1/2 cups milk (I used 2%)

Instructions

1. Instant Pot: Put all the ingredients in the first list into the Instant Pot. Cook for 45 minutes (manual, high pressure). Release steam using the valve on top.

2. Stovetop: When the soup is done, melt the butter in a saucepan. Whisk in the flour. Let the mixture cook for a minute or two to remove the floury taste. Whisk the milk, a little bit at a time, until you have a smooth, thickened sauce. Throw a little salt in there for good measure.

3. Together: Mix the creamy sauce with the soup in the instant pot. Voila! Mushroom Wild Rice Soup.

Prep Time: 15 Minutes

Cook Time: 25 Minutes

Servings: 3

Ingredients:

Crispy Tofu:

- 1 block of extra firm tofu (high protein tofu works really well in this recipe, if you can find it!)
- 2 tablespoons cornstarch
- 1 tablespoon soy sauce
- 2 tablespoons olive oil

Apricot Sauce:

- 1/3 cup apricot preserves
- 1 tablespoons soy sauce
- 1–2 tablespoons rice vinegar
- 1/2 teaspoon each cumin, paprika, and onion powder
- 1–2 cloves garlic, grated (2 for more garlic flavor, obviously)
- 1/4 teaspoon salt (more to taste)

Extras for Serving:

- toasted sesame oil to taste (I like about 1-2 tablespoons)
- chives and/or cilantro for topping
- steamed green beans
- cooked rice

Instructions

1. Cut the tofu block in half horizontally (like a hamburger). If using extra firm high protein tofu, it helps to cut it in half again horizontally. Press the water out of the tofu by wrapping it in paper towels and setting a few heavy books on top of it. Let it stay like that for a few minutes while you prep the sauce.
2. Whisk the sauce ingredients together.
3. Take each piece of tofu and gently pull it into small chunks with your hands (this just gives the tofu pieces a unique shape and texture that holds onto the sauce really well). Place the chunks in a bowl. Toss with soy sauce and a teaspoon or two of olive oil; then sprinkle with cornstarch and give it a few gentle tosses to coat.
4. In a nonstick skillet over medium high heat, heat the olive oil and then add the corn starched tofu. Leave it

undisturbed for a few minutes on each side, letting it get really nice and brown and crispy – this can take 10-15 minutes. Flip and repeat until the whole batch is browned and crispy.

5. While it's browning, you can start up your rice and/or sides!

6. Finally, add the sauce to the tofu and remove from heat – the pan will still be hot, so it'll be sizzle and smell really good from the garlic. The sauce will coat the tofu right away. heart eyes

7. Top with the green onions and/or cilantro, sesame seeds, and sesame oil. Serve with rice and green beans, and finish with more salt and lots of black pepper to taste. The tender crunch of the beans with the steamy rice and sticky tofu! SO good.

Prep Time: 3 Minutes

Cook Time: 12 Minutes

Servings: 18

Ingredients:

- 1 cup unsalted butter
- 1 cup lightly packed light brown sugar
- 1/2 cup heavy whipping cream
- 2 teaspoons flaky sea salt
- 10-ounce package miniature marshmallows (16 ounces for extra gooey!)
- 12-ounce box of Rice Krispies or crispy rice cereal (about 11–12 cups)

Instructions

1. Melt butter in a large pot over medium heat.
2. Add sugar and whipping cream; stir to incorporate. It will take a minute, but as it heats, you'll start to see a smooth, creamy caramel mixture form. Heat over medium-low heat for 5-7 minutes, until you have a

slightly thickened caramel sauce that coats the back of a spoon.

3. Remove from heat and stir in the salt. Taste and adjust for more salt if you want.

4. Add the marshmallows and stir until melted.

5. Stir in the cereal. Press mixture into a 9×13 pan. You might have a little bit of extra that doesn't fit in the pan – perfect for a little snack, if you ask me.

6. Cool slightly, cut into squares, and enjoy! You can eat these at room temperature, but I also love them in the refrigerator! They stay excellently tight, compact, and yet still soft and chewy as they thaw. For some reason that cold, crispy, buttery texture is just really enjoyable.

Prep Time: 10 Minutes

Cook Time: 15 Minutes

Servings: 4

Ingredients:

- Crispy Black Bean Tacos
- 1 (14 ounce) can of black beans, rinsed and drained
- 1/4-ish cup of your favorite salsa
- 1 tablespoon taco seasoning
- small flour tortillas
- olive oil or butter for frying

Cilantro Lime Sauce:

- 1/4 cup oil
- 1/4 cup water
- 1/2 cup chopped green onions
- 1/2 cup cilantro leaves
- 2 cloves garlic
- 1/2 teaspoon salt
- juice of 2 limes

- 1/2 cup sour cream (sub avocado to keep it dairy free / vegan)

Instructions

1. Blend all ingredients in the cilantro lime sauce until smooth-ish. Set aside.
2. In a food processor or chopper, blend the beans, salsa, and taco seasoning. Transfer to a skillet with a drizzle of oil and cook it up long enough to soften the flavors of the garlic and / or onions in the salsa. About 5 minutes is fine.
3. Spread a few tablespoons of black bean filling into a flour tortilla. Fold in half. Repeat until the filling is used up (about 6-8 tacos).
4. Heat some oil or butter in a skillet over medium heat. Fry in a skillet over medium heat, until crispy and golden brown. Dip in cilantro lime sauce. Serve with chips and salsa and a mid-week margarita. You're welcome.

11. Cauliflower Orange Gnocchi

Prep Time: 10 Minutes

Cook Time: 20 Minutes

Servings: 4

Ingredients:

- 1 package gnocchi (I use DeLallo)
- 2–3 tablespoons unsalted butter
- a medium-large head of cauliflower, cored and thinly sliced into bite-sized pieces on a mandoline (about 3 cups)
- 2 shallots, minced (about 1/3 cup)
- 1/4 – 1/2 cup heavy cream (see notes)
- 1/2 – 1 teaspoons red pepper flakes
- 1 1/2 teaspoons salt (more to taste)
- juice and zest of 1 orange (about 2 tablespoons of juice, zest to taste)
- chives for topping

Instructions

1. Cook the gnocchi according to package directions. Set aside.
2. Heat the butter over high heat in a large nonstick skillet. Add cauliflower, shallot, and cooked gnocchi; let it sit for a few minutes and then stir and repeat. You want the cauliflower and gnocchi to get browned, and the shallots to get soft.
3. Add in the cream, orange juice, red pepper flakes, and salt. Simmer for just a minute or two until desired consistency is reached – everything should be coated in a silky light sauce.
4. Serve immediately topped with fresh chives and orange zest. OH MY GOODNESS.

Prep Time: 10 Minutes

Cook Time: 35 Minutes

Servings: 4

Ingredients:

Cauliflower:

- 1 large head of cauliflower, cut into florets
- salt and olive oil
- 1 package taco seasoning (I like Siete brand)

Tostadas:

- 1 14–ounce can refried black beans (I like Amy's brand)
- 8–10 small corn tortillas (I like Mission street tacos tortillas)
- 1/4 cup of vegetable or canola oil
- cilantro
- pickled red onion
- queso (I like Queso Mama brand – the green chile variety)

Instructions

1. Preheat the oven to 425. Arrange the cauliflower florets on a baking sheet; drizzle with olive oil and sprinkle with salt. Roast for 25-30 minutes until browned and tender. Add taco seasoning directly to the pan; toss with the cauliflower using tongs until it's well coated. (You might not need a full taco seasoning packet for this.) Return to the oven for 5-10 minutes to get it nice, soft, and roasty-delicious.

2. Heat 1/4 cup of oil in a large skillet. You want the oil to be hot enough so that a speck of water dropped in will sizzle across the top. Add your tortillas to the oil, a few at a time depending on size, and fry for a few minutes on each side until golden brown and crispy. Place on a paper towel lined plate to remove excess oil, and repeat with remaining tortillas.

3. Top tortillas with warmed black beans, roasted cauliflower, cilantro, pickled onion, and warmed queso. Sprinkle with salt and lime juice as needed / wanted. OMG. Crunchy, creamy, tangy, and so darn good.

Prep Time: 10 Minutes

Cook Time: 20 Minutes

Servings: 4

Ingredients

- 1 block extra firm tofu
- 1 cup rice, uncooked
- 2 cups frozen shelled edamame
- 1 cucumber, finely diced
- 1 avocado, cut into chunks or slices
- 1 jalapeno, thinly sliced
- swish of neutral oil
- 1/2 cup teriyaki or savory-sweet Asian-inspired sauce (I used the store-bought Soy Vay brand – you could also make your own)
- 1/2 cup crunchy fried onions, crushed (like the kind you put on green bean casserole from the store!)
- spicy mayo

Instructions

1. Prep the tofu: Press the water out of the tofu.

2. Make the rice: Cook rice according to package directions.

3. Prep the edamame: Cook edamame according to package directions.

4. Cook the tofu: Cut the tofu into cubes. Heat a little oil over medium high heat. Add the tofu and fry until golden brown. Add about 1/4 to 1/3 cup of sauce – just enough to coat the tofu – and stir fry again until golden brown.

5. Serve: Assemble bowls with rice, tofu, more teriyaki sauce, edamame, cucumber, jalapeño, crunchy onions, and spicy mayo.

Prep Time: 10 Minutes

Cook Time: 30 Minutes

Servings: 8

Ingredients:

Salad:

- 1 cup Simple Nature Organic Quinoa, uncooked
- 5 ears sweet corn, cut off the cob
- 1 can Simply Nature Organic Black Beans, rinsed
- 1 package mini sweet peppers, sliced into small rings (about 2–3 cups)
- olive oil for cooking
- 1 cup chopped fresh cilantro

Dressing:

- 1/3 cup Burman's Mayonnaise
- 1/4 cup buttermilk
- 1 clove garlic, grated
- 1 teaspoon Stonemill Chili Powder
- 1/2 to 1 teaspoon salt
- juice and zest of two limes

- Pueblo Lindo Grated Cotija Cheese for topping

Instructions

Cook quinoa and prep ingredients.

1. Drizzle a generous amount of olive oil in a skillet and add the pepper rings. Cook over medium heat, stirring occasionally, for about 20 minutes or until very soft and roasty-looking. Squeeze a little lime juice in the pan to lift all the browned bits off the bottom of the pan when you're done! More flavor!

2. Whisk up the dressing ingredients. Taste and adjust. It's okay if it's super salty – it's going on a bunch of raw, unseasoned ingredients so we want it to have lots of flavor!

3. Toss ingredients or arrange in a bowl just before serving (quinoa, corn, beans, peppers, cilantro, and topped with dressing and cheese). Serve with grilled chicken, dip with chips, or on its own as a meal!

Prep Time: 10 Minutes

Cook Time: 15 Minutes

Servings: 11

Ingredients:

- 1/2 cup butter (I usually use salted), softened
- 1/2 cup packed light brown sugar
- 1/4 cup granulated sugar
- 1 egg
- 1 teaspoon vanilla extract
- 1 1/4 cups + 2 tablespoons flour, (if you have a scale, it should measure 7.3 ounces or 206 grams – if you do not have a scale, measure by spooning flour into the measuring cup and leveling it off)
- 3/4 teaspoon baking soda
- 1/2 teaspoon salt
- 1/2–3/4 cup freeze-dried strawberries
- 1/2 cup white chocolate chips

1. Preheat the oven to 350 degrees F.

2. Using a stand mixer or an electric hand mixer, combine the butter with the sugars until creamy.

3. Add the egg and vanilla; mix until just combined.

4. Add the flour, baking soda, and salt; mix until just combined.

5. Fold in the white chocolate chips. Crush the strawberry pieces gently by hand, not into powder but just into small chunks. Fold strawberry pieces into the dough.

6. Roll into balls (9-12 total) and bake on a parchment-lined baking sheet for 9-11 minutes depending on the size of your cookies. I usually do this in two batches. At 9-10 minutes, the cookies will be puffed up slightly; you'll want to let them sit out for a few minutes so they can sink back down and firm up into soft, dense, buttery, delicious little miracle cookies.

Prep Time: 10 Minutes

Cook Time: 30 Minutes

Servings: 4

Ingredients

- 3 tablespoons extra virgin olive oil
- 3 cloves garlic, smashed or thinly sliced
- one 28-ounce can whole peeled San Marzano tomatoes
- 1 teaspoon kosher salt
- Freshly ground black pepper to taste
- 4 cups vegetable or chicken broth
- 1/4 cup packed fresh basil, chopped or torn
- 2–3 cups dry bread, torn or cut into cubes

Instructions

1. Heat the olive oil in a large pot over medium heat. Add the garlic; sauté for 1 minute.
2. In a separate bowl, crush tomatoes by hand. Add them into the pot. Add salt and pepper. Partially cover and simmer over medium heat for about ten minutes.

3. Add the broth and basil; bring back to a simmer for
    another ten minutes.

4. Add the bread cubes; simmer for another ten minutes
    until the bread is soft. You can use a potato masher to
    further break down the bread to your desired texture.

5. Serve with Parmesan cheese, extra olive oil, and more
    fresh basil! Simplicity and top notch ingredients... it's
    just stunning.

Prep Time: 10 Minutes

Cook Time: 35 Minutes

Servings: 6

Ingredients:

- Roasted Vegetables
- 8 large carrots, peeled and chopped
- 3 golden potatoes, chopped
- 1 head of broccoli, cut into florets
- 1 head of cauliflower, cut into florets
- olive oil and salt
- Green Tahini
- 1/2 cup olive oil (mild tasting)
- 1/2 cup water
- 1/4 cup tahini
- a big bunch of cilantro and/or parsley
- 1 clove garlic
- squeeze of half a lemon (about 2 tablespoons)
- 1/2 teaspoon salt (more to taste – I like 3/4 teaspoon)

Optional Extras:

1. hard boiled eggs
2. avocados
3. chicken, tofu, any other protein

Instructions

1. Prep: Preheat the oven to 425 degrees.
2. Roasted Vegetables: Arrange your vegetables onto a few baking sheets lined with parchment (I keep each vegetable in its own little section). Toss with olive oil and salt. Roast for 25-30 minutes.
3. Sauce: While the veggies are roasting, blitz up your sauce in the food processor or blender.
4. Finish: Voila! Portion and save for the week! Serve with avocado or hard boiled eggs or... anything else that would make your lunch life amazing.

Prep Time: 5 Minutes

Cook Time: 25 Minutes

Servings: 4

Ingredients:

Tofu:

- 12 ounces extra firm tofu
- 1/2 cup soy sauce
- 1/4 cup rice vinegar
- 2 tablespoons agave
- 1 clove minced garlic

Bowls:

- white or brown rice
- carrots
- cucumbers
- avocado
- sesame seeds
- greens – I used microgreens
- pickled ginger
- soy sauce + wasabi for topping

- sriracha + mayo for the spicy mayo drizzle

Instructions

1. TOFU: Press the tofu to eliminate excess moisture. Cut into small cubes and marinate in the soy sauce, vinegar, agave, and garlic while you prep the veggies and other ingredients.
2. BOWLS: Prep all the veggies, rice, and toppings.
3. TOFU AGAIN: Heat a little bit of oil in a skillet. Drain off excess marinade and add tofu to the hot pan, shaking or stirring gently every so often to keep it from over-browning. When the tofu is browned, add to the bowls and serve.
4. ASSEMBLY: Divide the tofu, rice, and veggies into bowls. Top with soy sauce, spicy mayo, sesame seeds, and pickled ginger!

Prep Time: 15 Minutes

Cook Time: 30 Minutes

Servings: 3

Ingredients:

For the Sweet Garlic Lime Sauce:

- 3 cloves garlic
- 2 tablespoons rice vinegar
- 1/4 cup agave or brown sugar
- 1/4 cup fish sauce
- 1/3 cup lime juice
- 1/3 cup vegetable oil

For the Bowls:

- Rice Noodles
- Basil, Mint, and Cilantro (plz use all three – they're so good together!)
- Serrano Peppers
- Chopped Peanuts
- Avocado
- Veggies –> like carrots, bell peppers, and cucumbers

- Protein –> like shrimp, tofu, chicken (optional)

Instructions

1. SAUCE PREP: Pulse the sauce ingredients together in a blender or food processor.
2. NOODLE PREP: Cook your rice noodles by soaking them in cold water for about 30 minutes. When they're softened, transfer to a pot of boiling water for just a minute or two before quickly draining again. *This is my preferred method because it prevents them from getting overly sticky.
3. VEG PREP: Mince the herbs, slice the serranos, and peel or julienne cut the vegetables.
4. BOWL PREP: Toss the noodles (hot or cold! your choice, friend) with the sweet garlic lime sauce and all the other ingredients.

Prep Time: 10 Minutes

Cook Time: 30 Minutes

Servings: 6

Ingredients:

Tofu:

- 2 blocks of extra firm tofu
- 1–2 tablespoons cornstarch
- olive oil and salt
- 2 small (or 1 large) head of broccoli, cut into florets
- 2 red bell peppers, cut into strips
- 1 1/2 cups uncooked rice

Peanut Sauce:

- 1/2 cup peanut butter
- 1/3 cup low sodium soy sauce
- 2 tablespoons sesame oil (toasted or dark)
- 2 tablespoons rice vinegar
- 2 tablespoons sambal oelek or chili paste (this is where the "spicy" comes in, so add to taste)
- 2 tablespoons sugar, honey, or agave

- a small knob of fresh ginger, peeled
- a clove of fresh garlic, peeled
- 1/4 cup water

Instructions

1. Press liquid out of the tofu. Cube tofu and toss (gently) with the cornstarch until coated. Arrange on a baking sheet lined with parchment. Arrange broccoli and peppers on another baking sheet. Drizzle all with olive oil and salt. Roast both pans at 425 degrees for 20-30 minutes, until tofu is slightly crisped and broccoli is roasty and delicious.
2. While the tofu and broccoli are roasting, cook the rice.
3. Also, make the sauce by blending everything in a blender or food processor.
4. Serve tofu and broccoli with rice and a good drizzle of peanut sauce. YUM!

Prep Time: 10Minutes

Cook Time: 40Minutes

Servings: 6

Ingredients:

- 1 cup white or brown rice
- 1 head of cauliflower, chopped into florets
- 1 tablespoon olive oil
- 1 tablespoon taco seasoning, divided
- 1 14-ounce can of black beans, rinsed and drained
- 1/2 cup water
- 2 tomatoes, chopped
- half of a small onion, chopped
- juice of 2 limes + more wedges for serving
- 1/2 cup chopped fresh cilantro
- 2 ears of corn, kernels cut off the cob
- 1 avocado
- your favorite hot sauce for topping

Instructions

1. Rice: Cook the rice according to package directions.

2. Cauliflower: Heat the oven to 425 degrees. Toss the cauliflower florets with the olive oil and half of the taco seasoning. Sprinkle with salt and pepper. Roast for 20-25 minutes, tossing halfway through to prevent burning.

3. Beans: Combine the black beans, water, and remaining taco seasoning in a small saucepan. Bring to a low simmer. Mash the black beans with the back of a spoon until the mixture starts to get creamy. It should continue to thicken as it stays over medium low heat.

4. Pico: Toss the tomatoes, onion, limes, and cilantro together to make a pico de gallo. Season with salt.

5. The Moment of Glory: Build a big bowl with rice, refried beans, corn, pico de gallo, avocado, and a lime wedge. Top the bowl with your roasted cauliflower and add your hot sauce if you want!

Prep Time: 5 Minutes

Cook Time: 15 Minutes

Servings: 8

Ingredients

For the Summer Rolls:

- 8 rice paper wrappers
- a few torn leafy greens like rainbow chard
- 1 medium cucumber
- 1 medium bell pepper
- 2 medium carrots
- a handful of fresh mint
- a handful of fresh cilantro
- 1 avocado
- crushed peanuts for topping
- For the Peanut Sauce:
- 3 tablespoons canola oil
- 2 cloves garlic, peeled
- 2 tablespoons low sodium soy sauce (sub a gluten free tamari if you need to make the recipe GF)

- 1–2 tablespoons peanut butter
- 1 tablespoons water
- 1 tablespoons white distilled vinegar
- 1 tablespoons honey
- a big squeeze of lime juice
- a dash of fish sauce

Instructions

1. Place the ingredients for the peanut sauce in a food processor or blender. Pulse or blend until smooth.
2. Slice the cucumber, pepper, and carrots into thin strips about 3 inches long. Slice the avocado into pieces.
3. Soak one rice paper wrapper at a time into a bowl of warm-ish water for about 30 seconds. When you see or feel the wrapper getting loose and elastic-y, remove it from the water and set it on a damp towel. Pat it dry gently and dry your hands.
4. Arrange a few of the vegetables and herbs in the center of the wrapper horizontally, starting with the leafy greens and ending with the avocado. Fold the left and right sides towards the middle; fold the top flap over the vegetables, tuck everything in, and tightly roll it all

up. The wrapper will be very sticky and delicate so work carefully.

5. Cut the rolls in half and place on a serving platter (because if you're like me, they'll look better when they're cut in half and you're looking at the pretty vegetables inside instead of the wrap job). Drizzle with the sauce or dip in the sauce or both! I topped mine with crushed peanuts.

Prep Time: 15 Minutes

Cook Time: 30 Minutes

Servings: 6

Ingredients:

Rainbow Roll-Ups:

- carrots, cut into matchsticks
- cucumbers, cut into matchsticks
- red cabbage
- curry hummus
- cooked rice or quinoa (optional)
- peanuts and cilantro
- collard greens (leaf)

Peanut Sauce:

- 3/4 cup peanut butter
- 1/4 cup soy sauce (tamari or coconut aminos if gluten free)
- 1/4 cup rice vinegar
- 1/4 cup water
- 2 tablespoons honey

- 1 clove garlic

Instructions

1. Prep: Trim the stem/spine of the collard leaf – don't cut it completely off, but just cut it down so that it's nice and thin and pliable.
2. Roll: Arrange your fillings on the collard leaf. Fold the ends in and roll from front to back, trying to keep everything in there nice and tight. Watch video for a visual example.
3. Peanut Sauce: Run all the ingredients through a blender or food processor. Voila!

Prep Time: 10 Minutes

Cook Time: 30 Minutes

Servings: 6

Ingredients:

Simple Delicious Tomato Sauce:

- 2 tablespoons olive oil
- quarter of an onion, minced
- 1 large clove garlic, minced or thinly sliced
- 12 ounces DeLallo Passata Tomato Purée
- 1/2 cup broth or water
- torn basil
- 1/4 cup mascarpone cheese
- 1/2 teaspoon salt

Gnocchi:

- one 16-ounce package DeLallo Potato Gnocchi (I used shelf-stable gnocchi but frozen would also work)
- a handful of baby spinach
- 8 ounces fresh mozzarella cheese slices
- Parmesan cheese

Instructions

1. Make the sauce: Preheat oven to 400 degrees. Heat the olive oil over medium low heat. Add the onion and garlic; sauté until translucent and fragrant. Add passata and water or broth; bring to a low simmer. Add torn basil, mascarpone, and salt. YUM.

2. Bake it up: Add gnocchi and spinach. Stir to coat evenly with sauce. Top with mozzarella slices and a sprinkle of Parmesan. Bake for 15-20 minutes, until gooey and light golden brown on top. Serve with more basil. THE END. That's it. You're in heaven.

Prep Time: 10 Minutes

Cook Time: 40 Minutes

Servings: 6

Ingredients

The Maple-Mustard Dressing:

- 1/4 cup maple syrup
- 1/4 cup stone ground mustard
- 2–3 tablespoons soy sauce
- 2–3 tablespoons olive oil

The Bowl Stuff:

- 2 sweet potatoes, peeled and diced
- 2 blocks tempeh, cubed
- 3–4 cups kale, cut into small pieces
- 1 avocado
- 1/2 cup sauerkraut
- other toppings / add-ins: quinoa, crispy onions, pecans, apples, dried cranberries

Instructions

1. Make the dressing and marinate tempeh: Preheat the oven to 425 degrees. Shake dressing ingredients in a jar. Marinate the tempeh in about half of the dressing for about 30 minutes, or just while the oven heats up.

2. Roast tempeh and sweet potato: Place marinated tempeh (with marinade) on a baking sheet. Add sweet potatoes to the other half of the baking sheet. Drizzle with oil, sprinkle with salt, and roast for 25-30 minutes. When both are browned and roasted, toss the tempeh with a little more dressing so it soaks up lots of mapley-mustardy flavor.

3. Get the kale all yummy: Pro tip: place the kale in the same bowl that the marinated tempeh was in so it can grab onto all the leftover marinade in the bowl. Massage the kale with a little bit more dressing and the avocado, so the avocado kind of smashes into the dressing and makes it tender and a little bit creamy.

4. Toss and serve: Toss up the roasted tempeh, sweet potato, kale, sauerkraut, in a big bowl with any other extras that you like. I mean, RIGHT?! It's shockingly good.

Prep Time: 5 Minutes

Cook Time: 20 Minutes

Servings: 4

Ingredients

- The "Cheese" Powder:
- 1/2 cup nutritional yeast
- 6 tablespoons cornstarch
- 1 tablespoon onion powder
- 2 teaspoons garlic powder
- 1 tablespoon coarse salt
- 1/4 teaspoon turmeric and paprika (for color)

The Mac:

- 1/2 box elbow macaroni pasta
- 1 1/2 cups non-dairy milk (unsweetened almond milk, soy milk, or oat milk are my favorites)
- 3 tablespoons non-dairy butter
- teensy squeeze of lemon juice (optional)

Instructions

1. "Cheese" powder: Blend all cheese powder ingredients until you get a fine powder, about 30 seconds. Store this powder in a jar and this will be enough powder to make 3-4 future batches of vegan mac and cheese for ya!

2. Noodles: Cook macaroni according to package directions. Drain.

3. "Cheese" Sauce Magic: Pour milk + 3 tablespoons powder into a small saucepan. Whisk thoroughly and gently bring to a slow simmer until you are looking at a creamy, "cheesy" sauce.

4. Finish and Delight: Combine cheese sauce and cooked macaroni. Stir in your knob of butter. Finish to taste – I like just a tiny squeeze of lemon juice (not enough to taste like lemon, but just enough to wake the whole thing up), plus some freshly cracked black pepper. So creamy, so "cheesy", so yum.

Prep Time: 5 Minutes

Cook Time: 30 Minutes

Servings: 6

Ingredients:

- 2 tablespoons olive oil
- half of an onion, minced
- 2 carrots, peeled and minced
- 2 stalks celery, minced
- 3 cloves garlic, minced
- 2 tablespoons smoked paprika
- 1/2 teaspoon cumin
- 1/2 teaspoon turmeric
- 1 1/2 cups red lentils, rinsed
- 5 cups vegetable broth
- one 14-ounce can full-fat coconut milk
- a lot of fresh spinach, chopped
- 2 teaspoons kosher salt (more or less to taste)
- juice of one lemon
- garlic powder, onion powder, black pepper, or honey to taste

For serving (optional):

- crispy socca
- Or use a flatbread or naan for dipping

Instructions

1. Heat the olive oil in a large soup pot over medium heat. Add the onion, carrot, and celery; sauté until softened, about 5-10 minutes.
2. Add the garlic, spices, and lentils. Stir to combine and let it stay on the heat for just a minute to get the garlic smelling really good.
3. Add the broth. Bring to a simmer; place lid partially on the pot and simmer for 10 minutes, stirring once or twice during cooking time.
4. Add coconut milk, spinach, salt, lemon juice, and season to taste. (I like a little drizzle of honey, and a couple shakes of garlic powder, onion powder, and cranks of freshly ground black pepper.)
5. Serve with socca or some other flatbread for dipping and dunking. Wholesome, colorful, and SO yummy!

Prep Time: 5 Minutes

Cook Time: 30 Minutes

Servings: 4

Ingredients:

- 3 tablespoons butter
- 1 tablespoon oil
- 16 ounces mushrooms, stems removed, very thinly sliced (see FAQs)
- 1–2 shallots, minced
- 4 cloves garlic, thinly sliced
- 1/4 cup all-purpose flour
- 1/2 cup white wine (I used Chardonnay)
- 3 cups broth (see notes for a quick homemade MUSHROOM broth option with your stems)
- 1/2–1 cup heavy cream
- 1 teaspoon salt + more to taste
- freshly ground black pepper to taste
- just a bit of chopped fresh herbs

Instructions

1. Heat the butter and oil in a soup pot over medium high heat. Add the mushrooms and shallots; sauté for 10 minutes until soft, fragrant, and delicious. Add the garlic; sauté for 1-2 minutes.
2. Add the flour; stir to coat everything. It will be very thick and dry (see notes). Add the wine slowly, letting the mixture loosen up. Add the broth slowly, stirring to form a smooth-ish soup.
3. Add the cream and the salt, pepper, and herbs. Don't boil it, but if you can give it a little bit of time to just hang out over very low heat (or even off heat), that is ideal – the flavors get better with just a little time to sit. Then again, if you cannot wait (I often can't), it's also SO delicious right here, right now, right out of the pot.

Prep Time: 25Minutes

Cook Time: 35Minutes

Servings: 6

Ingredients:

- 1 tablespoon oil
- 5 cloves garlic, minced
- one 3-inch piece of ginger, peeled and cut into thin slices
- 3 stalks lemongrass, ends trimmed, outer layer peeled, and cut into bigger chunks
- 1–2 tablespoons roasted red chili paste
- 8 ounces fresh mushrooms, sliced
- 1 red bell pepper, thinly sliced
- 1 block of extra firm tofu, pressed and cut into small cubes
- 5–6 cups vegetable or chicken broth
- about 20 ounces full fat coconut milk (I like Aroy-D brand, and I use about 1.5 cans)
- 3 tablespoons fish sauce (more or less to taste)
- 3 tablespoons brown sugar

- juice and zest of 1-2 limes (to taste)

- salt to taste (about 1 teaspoon)

- lots of cilantro

- chili oil for serving

- rice for serving

Instructions

1. Heat the oil in a soup pot over medium heat. Add the garlic, ginger, and lemongrass; sauté for 3-5 minutes (but don't let the garlic brown – if it starts browning, remove from heat / turn the heat down).

2. When everything is soft-is and smells really nice, add the roasted red chili paste and sauté for 1-2 minutes. Add the mushrooms and red pepper (and any other veggies you like). Sauté for 3-5 minutes to get them sweating a bit, and then add the tofu and broth and bring to a simmer. Simmer for 10-15 minutes.

3. Add coconut milk, fish sauce, brown sugar, lime juice and zest, and salt. Stir in the cilantro. Taste and adjust till you get it just how you like it. Pull out the lemongrass chunks.

4. I like to ladle the soup over a shallow bowl filled halfway with rice – so the soup kind of goes on one side

and the rice on the other, with the coconuty broth spilling over into the rice a bit. Top it off with extra cilantro and chili oil. SO, SO GOOD.

Prep Time: 5 Minutes

Cook Time: 15 Minutes

Servings: 8

Ingredients:

- half a loaf of sourdough bread (THE BEST) but Tuscan bread or any kind of rustic loaf will work
- 1/2 cup olive oil
- 1 clove garlic, finely grated
- salt to taste
- freshly ground black pepper to taste

Instructions

1. Preheat oven to 400 degrees. Pull the bread into crouton-y sized chunks.
2. Combine the olive oil and garlic in a large bowl. Add bread and massage to work the oil in (some of the bread might crumble into tiny pieces, which provides great texture variety). Season thoroughly with salt and lots of pepper.

3. Bake for about 15 minutes, turning once so they get evenly browned. Cool on paper towels to absorb excess oil.

4. Use for dunking, dipping, and sopping up all that amazing soup; freeze your extras and re-toast in the oven for future soup-in!